31 Days to Fit

BY TERRI BONIN

TABLE OF CONTENTS

Introduction

I hate to sweat.

I can't diet.

I am no Jillian Michaels.

So if you are looking for a plan that will prepare you for *Iron Man*, this would only be the first teeny, tiny baby step-- *maybe.* I wrote <u>31 Days to Fit</u> as an answer to the question, "How do you get back into your jeans after each pregnancy?" The answer is NOT through a fast metabolism or good genes: no lanky body lurks around here. I am 5 feet tall, and I come from a long line of obesity. In fact, my large, second cousin dropped dead at a family reunion *while eating*! A special casket had to be built for him because he was too large for a standard casket. Yep, those are the genes that run through my blood!

When I was a teen my weight fluctuated by the day and I grew weary of it. I knew that if I did not change something permanently I would end up like my dear ol' second cousin. So after much nutritional study and prayer, I set up guidelines that keep my weight from fluctuating with or without exercise because quite honestly, I'm more likely to skip exercise than a meal. Fast forward close to half a lifetime from the season I established these guidelines to maintain a healthy weight. Since that time I have given birth to eleven healthy children, and by God's grace, I am still the *pre-children size* I was when my husband and I married, thanks to these guidelines. These ground rules for eating are simple, sustainable and achievable, and will work for you, too!

31 Days to Fit will work for anyone! It is basically a list of habits to keep for a lifetime revealed over 31 days. Throughout the book you will see a physical challenge as well as a spiritual challenge at the end of each post. I am challenging you in both areas because while our physical health is important, the state of our spirits is infinitely more important, so let's care for both.

Let's get started.

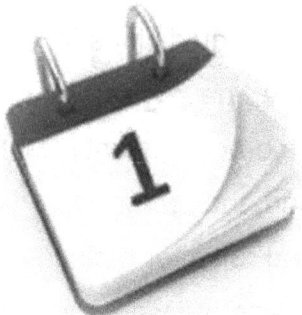

Day 1 – Why Bother?

Why do you want to be fit? Now, you may think this is a dumb question, but I want you to discover, for yourself, why YOU want to be fit. Do you need energy? Do you feel frumpy? Has your marriage lost its zing? Has the Lord convicted you to change some bad habits? If you don't own your reasons, you may lose focus. I want you to take a moment and think about your true motivation.

Now write a mission statement.

Do not write down a goal weight or a set a time frame for yourself to get into shape. I actually want you to throw away your scale. You may do this 31-day challenge a few times **before** it becomes a lifestyle. You are not to beat yourself up or get discouraged. This is a journey that will have ups and downs. You will go two steps forward and one step back in this journey, but it is OK. The condition of your body does NOT define who you are or equal your worth. You are valuable, beautiful and precious to your Creator no matter what shape you are in. So no self-condemning words along the way; this is going to be fun!

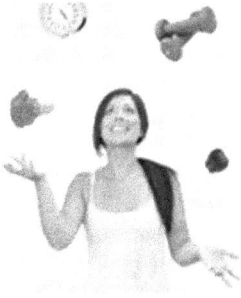

Physical Challenge:

If your life revolves around regular work hours, decide not to eat past 8pm from now on. Don't Eat Late. Do you struggle with this?

Spiritual Challenge:

Find your Bible. Buy a spiral and a pen. Ask the Lord to make you faithful.

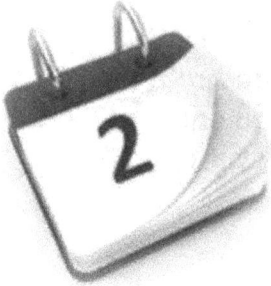

Day 2 - One Bad to the Bone Special Undercover Agent

You were created with a purpose. God prepared good works for you to do before the foundation of the earth was created: work only YOU can do. Just think, YOUR Creator was thinking about you even before you were born. I personally find this pretty cool. This speaks of love and hope. It breeds excitement. How can you know what YOUR special assignment is? What must you do to complete it?

There are two aspects to completing your purpose:

First, you must make an effort to hear His voice.

Second, you must be ready and willing to physically carry out whatever He whispers to you. This is not the time to suffer an ADD moment. You must be able to focus mentally to grow in your relationship with the Lord and you must have energy in order to carry out His assignment. This book is going to help you with both!

I remember one afternoon, as a young mom, I was lying on the couch in the middle of the day like a zombie, too tired to get my chores done or play with the kids. I knew that my tiredness came from the trashy food I had eaten that morning. I felt sad. I was sad because my bad choices were cheating my kids of a happy, energetic mom. I determined that day NOT to be a slave to anything that was going to steal from me.

Junk food was stealing my energy and sweet memory-making moments with my kids. I made the choice to take back my life.

Choose not to be a slave to anything that steals health and energy from you. Have you ever felt like a slave to a certain food item or food in general?

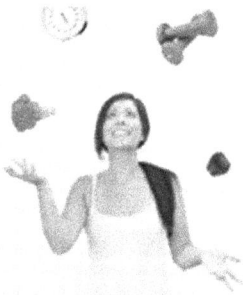

Physical Challenge:

Drink more water. Take half your body weight and turn it into ounces. That is how much water you should drink for energy. Caffeine depletes the choline in your brain, which affects your memory and ability to focus, so let water replace your caffeinated afternoon beverage. You will feel the

positive effects of increased energy and focus after the caffeine withdrawals subside. Sorry. I don't have a remedy for caffeine withdrawals; nor am I saying to NEVER drink caffeine; just no more heavy doses in the afternoon. And let's be honest, since you are probably NOT going to give up caffeine completely, buy the supplement MindWise by Young Living which supports cognitive function! It tastes yummy and gives a short term memory boost! I love it!

Spiritual Challenge:

Repent before the Lord for not taking the time to hear His voice. Seek Him by reading Psalm 1 and thinking about what it means.

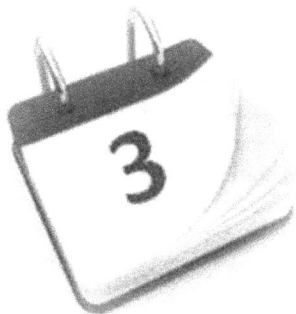

Day 3 – Shake it Up

Momentum is important when seeking real progress. If you want to see a significant difference at the end of our 31-day challenge, be sure you keep the past challenges as you add new ones. You are building habits that will benefit you for a lifetime. I recommend keeping a visible list of your new habits until they are truly habits. Each day add the new challenge to the list and review the previous. Don't beat yourself up if you mess up. Every second is a new start. You are not on a diet; you are simply changing a few lifestyle habits so that your weight will stop fluctuating and you will have more energy to complete the tasks that are truly important to you. So just keep moving forward and don't sit down in defeat, no matter how bad you mess up these challenges.

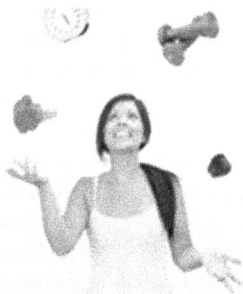

Physical Challenge: Commit to taking the stairs instead of the elevator, and DO IT! You will elevate your heart rate and speed up your metabolism for a

calorie burning effect. Your legs will also be strengthened in the process.

Spiritual Challenge: Open your Bible to Proverbs. It's in the middle. Now read the chapter of Proverbs that coincides with the day of the month aloud to your children over a healthy breakfast. Commit to reading a portion of scripture aloud to your children each day while they live at home. Make it fun! Stay committed.

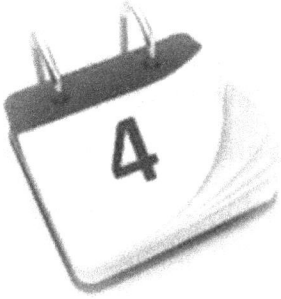

Day 4 – Them Boots Weren't Made for Walking

You have a few good habits in place. *Woo Hoo!* Good job! You are going to bed without a heavy meal sitting on your stomach--This means you should be waking up brighter. You are drinking more water, which means you should have energy throughout the day, and you are taking the stairs instead of the elevator, which gives you an extra bounce in your step. You are reading your Bible daily and seeking insight into your special assignments.

Today, I want you to find your tennis shoes. If you need to buy new ones, do so, because a good pair of walking shoes will make exercising much easier. If you don't wear good shoes you will ultimately hurt your back and knees, which will make an active life harder.

When I was *very* pregnant with our sixth child, my husband and I ventured out to a car show on one of our dates. I waddled around the stadium thinking I was going to DIE my back hurt so bad. *(I can be dramatic. Besides, I was pregnant! A little drama is to be expected.)* My sweet husband understood my misery and took me straight to a specialty shoe store he had heard a friend talking about. Within an hour my feet donned new tennis shoes with solid soles and a coil under each heel. I could not BELIEVE the difference those shoes made in the way I felt, even in my third trimester of pregnancy. Good walking shoes allowed me to exercise all the way to the end of that pregnancy.

Case inpoint: Wear good walking shoes.

Do you walk? If so, what are your favorite walking shoes?

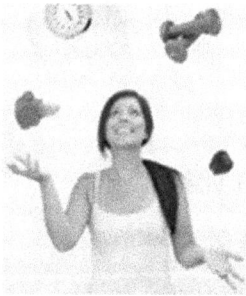

Physical Challenge: Schedule a daily walk (or three days a week, if that's what fits your schedule.) I like to walk 2 miles in the evenings when I walk. If you don't want to track the miles, you can simply set a timer and walk for 45 minutes. Just walk and walk briskly. This one change in your lifestyle could trim many pounds off your body! Try it for at least a year. If you find that your joints and ligaments hurt when you walk, then take the supplement AgilEase by Young Living. This one makes

a HUGE difference in my ligaments! It takes away pain from old injuries and allows me to walk pain free.

Spiritual Challenge: The Lord has many names. Look them up and learn to pray using the specific names of God. Jehovah Ezer is the God who helps. Call on Jehovah Ezer to help you keep these healthy habits. Prayer will make a world of difference in combating bad habits.

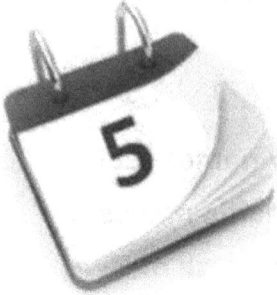

Day 5 - One Step at a Time

I have been blessed with eleven amazing children, but I didn't wake up one day and just have a house full of beautiful bouncing babies. God built our family slowly, one child at a time. He stretched my husband and me along the way, teaching us to invest our time and energy into these souls. It's a good thing God did not give us all eleven children at once; we would have been overwhelmed and discouraged with the insurmountable task of raising our children properly. God, in His wisdom, grows us one step at a time. Likewise, build your new healthy habits one step at a time, giving yourself time to adjust and grow with these changes. Slow and steady gets the job done more thoroughly than a crash diet. Today is your Five Good Habits marker. You are building momentum.

Here are some important tips to remember:
1) Don't eat late.
2) Drink more water.
3) Commit to taking the stairs instead of the elevator.

4) Schedule a brisk walk 30-45 minutes long, at least 3 times a week.

5) Eat a salad everyday.

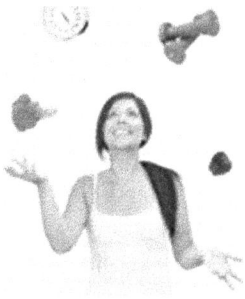

Physical Challenge: Eat more salad. Eat one every day! Make sure your salad consists mostly of vegetables and not chips, beans, meat and cheese. (Or make yourself a mini vegetable tray and crunch away.)

Spiritual Challenge: Get up thirty minutes earlier than usual to spend time reading your Bible and journaling your prayers. This practice will strengthen and encourage your spirit, which is more important than any physical habit we add. You can do it!

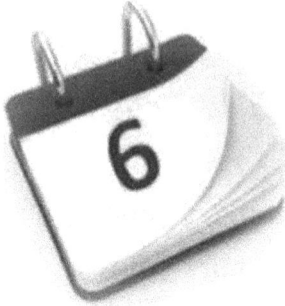

Day 6 - Don't Multi-task

I decided to blanket train my ten-month-old while writing today's entry. It didn't go so well. In fact, it took me ten minutes to realize writing and child training don't make good companions. After setting my laptop down three times before completing one coherent thought, I aborted the blanket-training mission and set the little explorer free. Now, my toddler's toys lay abandoned while she commences to eat the books in the basket by my chair. The life lesson I gather from this is that multitasking is not always a productive choice and my writing needs to take place while she sleeps. Another multitasking combo that can be disastrous is eating and watching a show at the same time. Don't do it. You will mindlessly eat enough food for three people and regret it later.

Do you struggle with mindless eating?

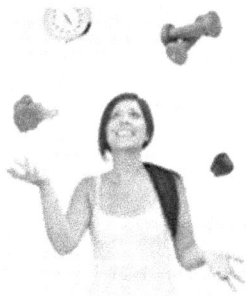

Physical Challenge: Read food labels. An extra 100 calories a day for one year can pack an added ten pounds on your body. That is just a big bite or two! Stay aware of how much you put into your mouth and make your snacks nutrient packed so your cells will be satisfied. Dried Wolfberries by Young Living are one of my favorite snacks to grab when I need to munch. They are filled with fiber, nutrients and keep my blood sugar balanced, three great benefits for the body. Whatever snack you choose, stay aware of the recommended serving sizes on all prepared food.

Spiritual Challenge: Memorize and meditate on Colossians 3:20, "Whatever you do, work at it with all your heart as working for the Lord and not for men."

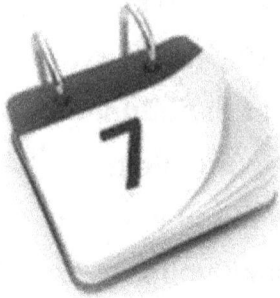

Day 7 - Rest

You're off today. Enjoy yourself, but not to the point of regret!

"This is the day the Lord has made, let us rejoice and be glad in it." Psalms 118:24

See you tomorrow!

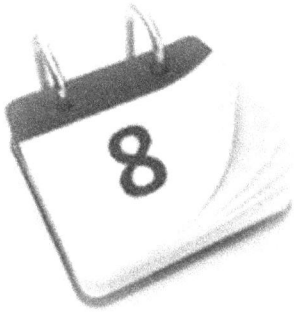

Day 8 - Multitask

No, I'm not schizophrenic. I realize I told you *not* to multitask on Day 6, but there's a time for almost everything under the sun and now is the time to multitask. On day five I challenged you to schedule a daily brisk walk. This heart pumping, arm-swinging exercise will clear the cobwebs from your cranium like none other. This is a great time to pray for each of your kids; cover your husband in petitions; and spill all your troubles before the Lord. It's energizing to the body and healing to the soul.

I talk aloud to Jesus while I walk---always have. Before Bluetooths were apart of our society, I'm sure I looked like a nut talking to myself, but I didn't care because my soul was revived. I highly recommend praying and walking at the same time. The serotonin that is pumped into your brain while you walk will give you a mental lift and ward off depression, also. This is a GREAT time to multitask.

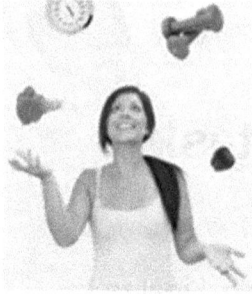

Physical Challenge: Learn to snack on frozen berries. Frozen fruit can be so satisfying to your taste buds while your cells are being fed immune boosting antioxidants. Frozen fruit is also a great source of fiber, so it's great for your intestines too. Buy a bag of organic mixed berries at the grocery store this week and snack away!

Spiritual Challenge: Fill your soul with some good praise music. Load it onto your phone and in your car. Your spirit will be encouraged and strengthened as you worship the Lord.

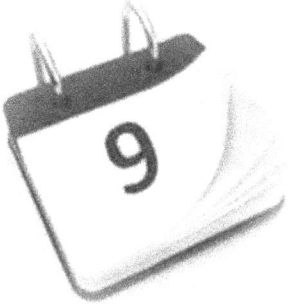

Day 9 - The Kiss of Death

I'm a hypocriteljust thought you would want to know. While the aroma of brownies waft around my nose, I am going to tell you how bad sugar is for you. Sugar is addictive and fattening. It is *impossible* to eat a lot of sugar regularly and be healthy. Sugar pounds on your thyroid, alters your mood and messes with your pancreasIIts only GOOD attribute is that it TASTES YUMMY.

At one point in my life, I fasted from sugar for seven solid years. I needed to take a break from the seducing fare because I was addicted and did not know how to eat only one brownie. I had to completely restrain myself. With me, it was ALL or NOTHING...NO dessert or HALF THE CAKE. I had headaches, fluctuating weight, and no sense of well being. Once I "got off of it", I was scared to death of the tempting sweets, unsure if self-control would always be an issue. I wondered if I would ever be the master and sugar the slave.

Thankfully, many years have passed, and I can eat sugar in moderation.

I do not need to give you an apologetic convincing you to cut down on sugar.

*You know it alters your hormones.

*You know it messes with your whole chemistry.

*You know it makes you fat.

So what are you waiting for? If you are addicted to sugar, begin a sugar fast; but get ready for the withdrawals since your body has become dependent. Sugar should be a once in awhile thing in your home. Look into buying Stevia extract. I buy the Sweet Leaf brand. Stevia is a great alternative to other health zapping options. I add it to sparkling water and unsweetened tea. Your body will thank you, and you will ultimately trim off many pounds with this little trick.

My kids whine sometimes because we are not normal and our pantry is not stocked with the sugary treats our neighbors have. Other times they thank me, because deep down, they know that eating sugar everyday rots teeth, attributes to diabetes, acne, and other major inconveniences. Get the sugar in your life under control.

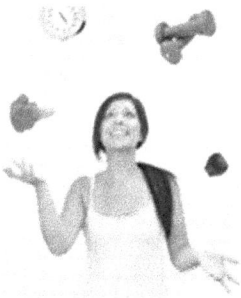

Physical Challenge: Throw away all white sugar in your home. Substitute raw, unbleached sugar in its place when baking for your kids. Guard your mouth from eating sugar more than twice a week if you truly desire a trim figure. The Trim Healthy Mama cookbook is full of yummy non-fattening desserts if you enjoy cooking. If not, then try sweetening your tea, carbonated water and plain yogurt with stevia extract! You'll be surprised how satisfying it is. Make your healthy sweet tooth options easily accessible, easily prepared, and easily sustainable. Sweet treats don't have to be fattening or complicated.

Spiritual Challenge: Memorize 2 Corinthians 4: 16-18, "Therefore we do not lose heart. Though our outer nature is wasting away, our inner nature is being renewed day by day. For this slight momentary affliction is preparing for us an eternal weight of glory beyond all comparison, as we look not to the things that are seen, but to the things that are unseen. For the

things that are seen are transient, but the things that are unseen are eternal."

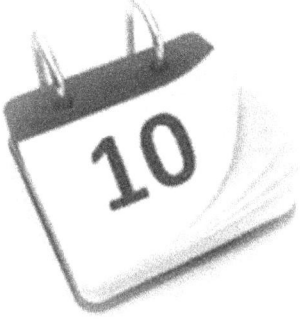

Day 10 - No Thank You and Then Some

The waiter returned with the dessert tray, and I cordially declined the delicacies while keeping my eye on the double decker death-by-chocolate fifteen layer cake. My sweet knowing husband ordered one for himself with a scoop of ice cream and two spoons.

I LOVE THAT MAN.

You see, he has learned. Dessert **does not** count for me, if I don't order it.

Seriously.

Just share.

Make it a lifetime habit to split a dessert rather than ordering your own and you will save tens of thousands of calories and fat grams within one year! and it's not that big of a sacrifice!

On this same note, I purchased little 8 oz Corelle bowls for ice cream and cereal at home. It's easy to share at a restaurant, but it's different at home. Everyone wants their own! And most of the pretty bowls that I like to buy are just too big for a single serving. An actual serving size looks like a small dollop in a Texas-sized dish, so I found some small bowls that make eating the suggested serving size less defeating. In summary: share a dessert when you are out to eat, and make sure the size of your dishes isn't undermining your efforts at home.

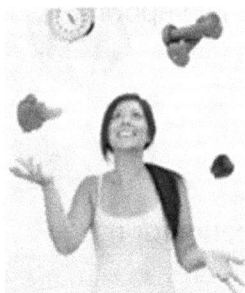

Physical Challenge: Lift arm weights 4 days a week. I like to do 3 sets of 20 reps of random arm exercises with 10 pound weights about 4 times a week or my arms begin to look like legs for lack of exercise, so I think. I keep the weights in my bathroom and do them usually when I'm getting dressed for bed because it's convenient. (Like I said on Day 1, I'm no Jillian Michaels.)

Spiritual Challenge: Are you still reading a chapter from Proverbs to your kids each morning? Training your kids in the Lord is WAY MORE IMPORTANT than any physical challenge I am giving you. Continue to

enjoy shaping their souls while they live under your roof.

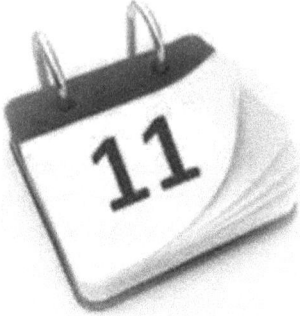

Day 11 - Splat

This is confession time--I broke one of my "guidelines" last night.

I ate late!

The buttery smell of popcorn lured me into the kitchen, while my kids' chatty conversation held me hostage. Before I knew it, I was stuffing my face and talking with my mouth full. Yes, I could have visited with my offspring and abstained from the crunchy corn, but an occasional late night snack won't break the scale (especially since I threw mine away a long time ago).

So this is my point: This book contains guidelines to follow INOT rules to be broken. If the majority of the time, you live by these guidelines, you will feel more energetic, be able to button your jeans without doing the worm dance on the bed, and be freed from ever having to crash diet before a high school reunion. So enjoy your stable weight, and view these guidelines as your new best friends, not your taskmaster.

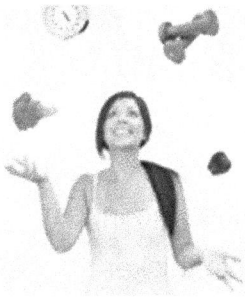

Physical Challenge: Get rid of all your fat and skinny clothes. Trim your closet down as your body settles into its natural weight. And do not compare your natural weight to someone else's. God made us each uniquely different sizes. Enjoy the healthy body He gave you and do not obsess over a certain size. If you NEED to shed a size or two, these tips should make it happen.

Listen to fun music and drink hot herbal tea while you do this activity.

Spiritual Challenge: Write a note of encouragement to someone you know who is having a hard time. Include a scripture promise and know that your promise as you do this is Proverbs 11:2, "He who refreshes others will himself be refreshed." When I was a young mom, sometimes at my wits end with 3 children 3-years-old and under, I began this practice. I would sit down when I felt like throwing an, "I've got poopy diapers everywhere pity party," and write notes of encouragement to other people in order to refocus myself AWAY from myself. It works.

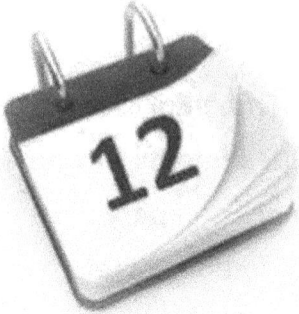

Day 12 - Get Real

Studies prove that people who ingest artificial sweeteners have thicker waists than those who don't. I drank diet drinks for YEARS and I can attest to the fact that my weight fluctuated by ten pounds regularly back then. The substance is called artificial because it IS NOT REAL! Your body is made up of the elements of the earth and it NEEDS those natural elements in order to function at peak performance. It CRAVES those natural elements. When an artificial ingredient is ingested, the body reacts by bloating. It reacts because it wants to protect you. Do your research.

Studies also link various diseases to different artificial sweeteners and it is proven that artificial sweeteners do not keep the blood sugar down. The fake sugars actually raise blood glucose in lab rats. So basically they have NOTHING good to offer. Ignorance is not bliss concerning anything artificial.

The information is easy to find.

http://articles.mercola.com/sites/articles/archive/2010/09/15
/aspartame-side-effects.aspx

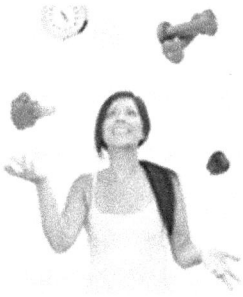

Physical Challenge: Throw away anything in your house with artificial sweeteners in it and toss all your little packets, too. Artificial sweeteners cause cravings that will keep you pudgy.

Spiritual Challenge: Speaking of sugar: Be extra sweet to your honey today. Speak to him in his love language and then some. Be happy because you probably already feel more confident in your lingerie. And yes, I am fully aware that I wrote this under the Spiritual Challenge. Blessing your husband when you don't feel like it takes spiritual strength and reaps spiritual rewards. Have fun! You are a wonderful creation, no matter what size you are! Your relationship is worth it! For more tips like this one, read my two marriage books: 14 Days to Ignite Your Marriage, and Drops of Pleasure: A Guide to Great Sex with Essential Oils.

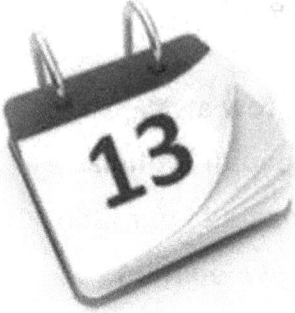

Day 13 - Fill 'er Up

Everyone is fat. Look around. It's ALMOST true. It seems like the population splits into two physical categories: fat or buff. Well, I don't want to be fat, and I do not have time to spend hours upon hours at the gym working out in order to be buff. So what is the solution?

Two little words: Portion. Control.

We are revisiting this one because it's crucial to your success for non fluctuating weight. In our family, portion control comes pretty easily most of the time. Everything is split twelve ways, so we all are forced to eat the recommended serving size, much to some individuals' dismay.

The other day I was preparing a special dinner for my honey and our little chickens (that's what we call our children).

Ice cream with homemade praline sauce was to be the finale after the meal.

At the grocery store, I was meticulously reading the back of ice cream cartons when my ready-to-go daughter hurried me with, "Just grab three big cartons. We'll eat it all."

Laughing, I reminded her that the ice cream was the dessert, NOT the main course and we only needed enough for this one meal. "But Mooooommmmm! How am I going to eat three bowls if you only buy ONE carton?"

"Isn't that the point, sweetie?" Seriously.

Overeating is the American way, and it has made us one of the fattest countries in the world. When you only eat the serving size, you will find yourself eating several small meals a day, which will keep your metabolism revved up and your tummy trim. When you are used to eating second helpings at each meal it's HARD to push back from the table,but you have to decide what you want more: the food or the figure? Pushing back from the table will help your body in many ways. Make it happen. You can do it!

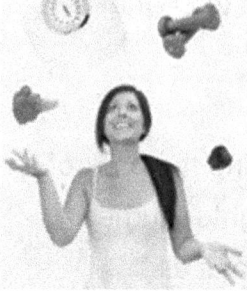

Physical Challenge: Determine to eat only the recommended serving size at each meal. You will feel hungry at first while your stretched out stomach adjusts, but you will feel better in the long run.

Spiritual Challenge: Write John 17:3 on an index card and tape it to your kids' bathroom mirror. "And this is eternal life: that they know You, the only true God, and Jesus Christ, whom you have sent." I love this one! My little ones learn it when they are 4!

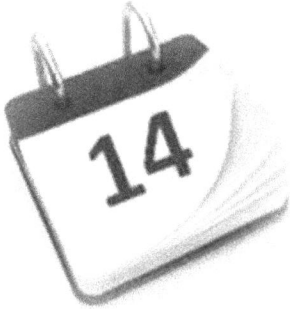

Day 14 - Rest

You have permission to think about NONE OF THIS today! This day of rest will empower you for long term success. Rest!

Enjoy!

See you tomorrow!

Matthew 11:28-29 *"$Come to me, all who labor and are heavy laden, and I will give you rest. Take my yoke upon you and learn from me, for I am gentle and lowly in heart, and you will find rest for your souls. For my yoke is easy, and my burden is light."*

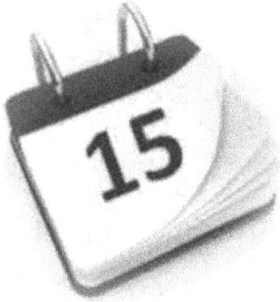

Day 15 - The Skinny on Skinny

So do you feel like you NEED to shed a size or two, but your body is hanging on to every last pound? This tip will kick it into gear. However, it's seriously simple in theory and painfully hard in application. Here it is: Give up flour. Yep. Those three little words hold the secret to the size of your waist.

Give. Up. Flour.

Think about everything you eat that has flour in it: bread, tortillas, gravy, cake, pastries, bagels, pasta, waffles, pizza, wheat-based cerealsII could go on. Grain flour becomes a sticky paste in the gut which flattens the villi in the intestines, which in turn makes it impossible to absorb nutrients. This means your brain will always be crying for more food because it is looking for nutrients but is only getting calories, which it stores as fat.

If you rid your lifestyle of flour, you will have more energy and clarity of mind. I personally don't care to live without flour my whole life, so initially I did a 40 day cleanse from it, and now I have flour-based products occasionally. I can *always* feel the difference in my energy level when I eat flour, so it's not that tempting to me anymore.

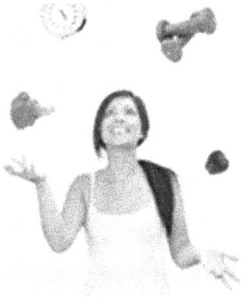

Physical Challenge: Give up grain flour for 40 days as a test. I believe you will feel more energetic and never go back to eating it daily.

Spiritual Challenge: Consider a weekly fast of some type. We are called to fast and pray, so pick one day a week and make it a habit. I like the book Fasting by Jentezen Franklin. He gives clear insight into the importance of fasting. I heard someone say once, "There are just some things I want more than I want food!" I couldn't agree more! This is what fasting is about. Read the book and gain insight.

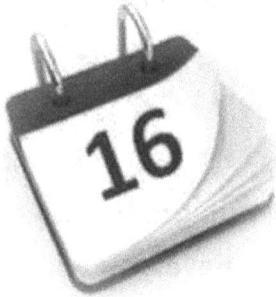

Day 16 - Sabotaged

My toddler can empty the kitchen cabinets faster than a speeding bullet. Chubby hands swiftly pull boxes of tea and plastic containers into a giant disarray of clutter onto the floor usually seconds before Daddy gets home.

I could put child locks on each of the lower doors, but that would be no fun for our adventurer, and thankfully, Daddy sees the strewn items as a sign of life being lived to the fullest.

My little cherub's creativity grows while exploring shapes, textures and sounds by banging plastics together and onto the tile.

My kitchen not only provides physical nourishment through healthy food for my family, but it is a playground for each of my kids in the toddler stage.

In my future, there will be a day when all the containers stay neatly in the cabinets because no toddler scales the floor.

Until then, I will celebrate life and recognize the little piece of the bigger picture growing in front of my eyes, and overlook the fact that my tot sabotages ALL my kitchen cleaning efforts.

You are on a journey to good health.

When you feel like other people are sabotaging your habits, don't get frustrated.

Find something to be thankful for and just do the best you can. This is not a race—this is a lifestyle.

The souls of people are more important than any of our goals.

Romans 14:20, "Do not destroy the work of God for the sake of food!" This is a journey, not a race...If you go two steps forward and one step back, it's OK.

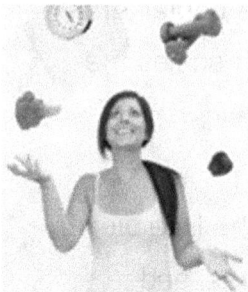

Physical Challenge: Take vitamins and supplements. Our food is so depleted of nutrients there is no way you are getting everything you need simply by eating. Start with a good multivitamin, an Omega fish oil and an enzyme. I take Young Living supplements because I trust their Seed to Seal quality promise and their products WORK in my body! If you need supplements, try these. My daily vitamin regimen right now consists of Master Formula, Sulfurzyme, AgilEase, Thyromin, EndoGlze, Ningxia Red and MindWise. I also love and sometimes take Essentialzyme, Digest and Cleanse and Omegagize also by Young Living. Peruse their benefits on my website justalittledrop.com or view the educational videos on dropsofjoy.com

Spiritual Challenge: Start a List of Thankfulness in your spiral. Count your blessings and keep the list growing.

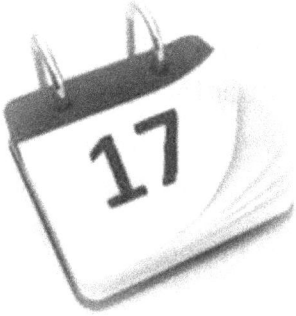

Day 17 - Sleep

Tucked away and deeply enjoying my dreamland, something in my subconscious whispered to another part of my brain, "YOU'RE GOING TO BE LATE!" Like a dead man coming to life, I bolt up leaving my dreamlandl far-far away.

I overslept.

The book I was reading last night was just too good to put down and now my whole body protests. With a mere ten minutes to dress and drive to the restaurant, I text my friend that I am running five minutes late for our coffee date. Five minutes...Ha!

I will be a sight at breakfast.

Throwing on my clothes, I pick up my now fussing baby, nurse her while I brush my bed-head and apply a scant amount of make-up.

Running down the hall, still nursing the tot, I wake up my oldest daughter, lay the hopefully full baby in bed with her and whisper instructions to my teen. I tuck them snugly under the downy comforter and fly out the door to meet my friend for coffee.

After my short night, coffee is certainly what I need, right?

Well let's break it down. I stayed up too late, pushing the limit on my adrenal glands; then I awoke with an abrupt start going from a dead sleep to running around the house 0-50 mph within seconds, taxing my adrenal glands more.

Caffeine will make up for the lack of sleep last night, and sugar will charge me in the afternoon.

Good choices? NOT!

But this is an all too common scenario. Studies show that I if I continue this lifestyle, I will be ten pounds heavier in a few months because of the extra fuel I will need to keep me awake. Sleeping is just as important as eating right and exercising.

The body goes into repair mode during the down hours, restoring through the night whatever calls for repair. This is one reason it is important NOT to go to bed with a stomach full of food. Your body needs to regenerate throughout the night, NOT digest. The proper amount of sleep is essential for total health. Value your shut-eye. http://www.mayoclinic.com/health/sleep-and-weight-gain/AN02178

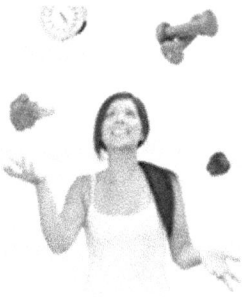

Physical Challenge: Turn the light off at a decent hour. If you are committed to the physical challenge on Day 1, you will want to go to sleep, so you don't have to listen to your stomach growl. Your body will reward you with vibrant energy in the morning. If it does not reward you, keep building these habits. Your body will eventually catch up with you. If you have trouble falling asleep, rub the essential oil blend Tranquil on your neck and temples. Diffuse lavender by your bed. You can even drink a few drops of Young Living's Vitality Lavender. I do this often! Using essential oils to help you sleep will not leave you groggy in the morning like medicinal sleep aids. You will sleep deep and wake up fresh.

Spiritual Challenge: Write Psalms 4:8 on an index card and teach it to your kids. "In peace I will both lie down

and sleep; for you alone, O Lord, make me dwell in safety."

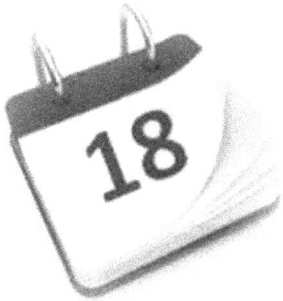

Day 18- But I Can't Sleep

There's a reason.

First, we can probably blame Thomas Edison for this problem. But regardless of who started it, we must take responsibility for the switch—and turn it off. Yesterday, you learned that leaving the light on late could make you fat. Today it gets worse—sorry.

Leaving that darn light on too late can cause hormonal imbalances in your body that will disrupt your daily life, causing you to cry at the most inconvenient times and snap impatiently at other times. This hormonal imbalance causes your highs to almost disappear and your lows to hang around, yet your body will resist sleep.

Let me explain!

Serotonin is the happy hormone and melatonin is the sleepy hormone. They are the opposite sides of the same wheel. If one side is flat the other will not work correctly either. So how can you put air back in your hormonal tire for a smoother ride?

Start with aerobic exercise. If you are doing this challenge correctly, you should already be experiencing a serotonin high when you walk each day. If you are walking long and hard, your sleep should not be so elusive. Before you try expensive sleep disorder testing for your sagging eye lids, make sure your lifestyle welcomes sleep naturally.

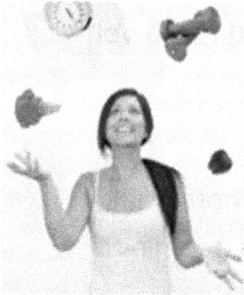

Physical Challenge: Around 3pm most bodies scream for a nap or a snack, but a snack is usually the only option. If this is true for you, then eat the following recipe each day when your body sags. We can thank the Trim Healthy Mama's for this treat! Combine equal parts light cottage cheese and organic mixed berries with a few squirts of stevia in a Vitamix and blend thoroughly. It's SO GOOD you'll feel like you're eating a fattening dessert. I sprinkle dark chocolate chips on mine and mmmm.. I'm in love. The berries have fat burning properties that work on the tummy, which is great because I HATE SIT-UPS! If you have stubborn pounds to lose, I think you'll find this one recipe quite helpful.

Spiritual Challenge: "It is vain for you to rise up early, To retire late, To eat the bread of painful labors; For He gives to His beloved even in his sleep," Psalm 127:2...Think about it.

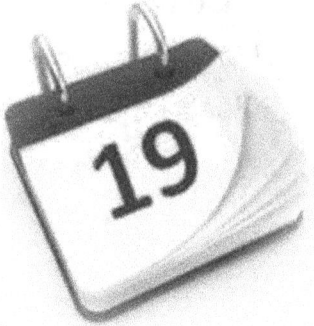

Day 19- Eat for Life

I answered the door and the picture of health greeted me: tall, brawn, bulging muscles, covered with smooth, young skin. A long-time friend of the family stopped by for a very sad meeting. He had stage 4 colon cancer. His physique hid the ruins that lived beneath.

My heart broke.

He was coming to us for instructionlfor help. Reversing the damage at that point in the game would have taken drastic measuresl including a miracle. Neither happened and we lost our friend a few months later. His young family was left without a daddy, a bride without her husband.

I cannot stress enough to you the importance of eating real, live, natural fiber. Fiber drinks are gross both coming and going. Just take care of it the way our Creator intendedl and eat fibrous foods. We cannot improve upon what God created. Laxatives will move things out with many cramps, but they will not exercise and brush the sides of your intestines the way fruits and vegetable will. If you must douse everything in dip to get you started, do whatever it takes and get raw, fresh fruits and vegetables inside your body. This will also give you energy.

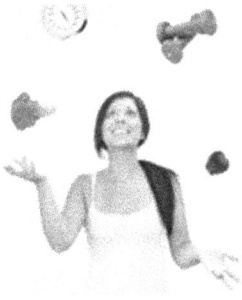

Physical Challenge: Eat an apple a day. There is quite a bit of truth to the old adage, "An apple a day keeps the doctor away." Apples are known for curing asthma, clearing acne, healing constipation and the list goes on. Eat them and buy them for your children. Please. However, if you have trouble implementing the apple a day, then take the intestinal Cleansing Trio by Young Living. It's absolutely elite with its ingredients and therapeutic essential oils. Regardless of what you do for your colon, be good to it! It requires fiber to get the waste out properly.

Spiritual Challenge: Are you getting alone with your Bible and your journal daily? If you have not already written each verse down that I have given you, do it now. Tell the Lord everything you are thankful for and then tell Him your needs in your journal.

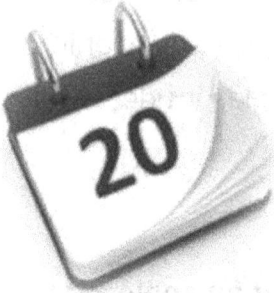

Day 20 - Stuffing your Mouth but Starving to Death

Propped up at the kitchen bar, my sticky-faced, gooey-handed three-year-old asked for a THIRD peanut butter and jelly sandwich. He had been eating an unusual amount lately.

I shrugged it off as he was growing.

But the truth was that my usually vibrant blonde headed boy had glassy eyes, low energy, and sores on his mouth-- and had for about a month. It dawned on me when he made the request for another sandwich, that his new eating frenzy completely paralleled his sluggish side effects.

A light flipped on in my brain, the problem was exposed and laid naked.

How could I have missed it?

I felt like a complete idiot and bad mother all in one fell swoop for being so slow to recognize it. My child was allergic to the wheat, the gluten or the peanut butter. I discussed my discovery with my husband and to make it easier on our little one, the whole family gave up the suspected items for a time as a test.

Within the first three days, my tot's eyes cleared, his vibrant energy returned and his mouth began to heal. Sometimes our bodies seem to crave that which will hurt us.

Why? Good question.

But it happens, so you should be fully aware that just because your body is CRAVING something DOES NOT MEAN YOU NEED IT.

Sometimes when a body needs protein, it will crave sugar. When you think you are craving ice cream, stop and think. What are the elements in ice cream your body might be wanting? It could be that you need some sugar energy (go for a complex carbohydrate not a simple carbohydrate), or protein from the milk for growth. The chemistry in your body crying out for certain elements, does not know about your favorite ice cream. Your habits simply rush you into a "quick fix."

Your body needs specific nutrients and if you eat a bowl of ice cream chalk full of calories and fat, and devoid of nutrition, your body will not be satisfied and you will have to eat something else too.

Thus obesity marries malnutrition.

They go hand in hand. People overeat trying to fill their nutritional needs, but the specific needs do not get met, so they eat and eat. Consider why you overeat. Is your body screaming for more vitamins, minerals and fish oils? Make **every** bite count and evaluate your cravings.

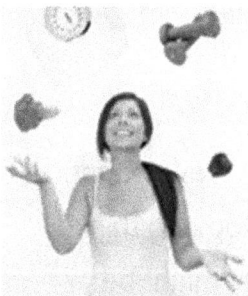

Physical Challenge: Be a detective. Listen to your body. Notice when you crave a specific food. Deduct what your body might really be saying. Choose wisely. Eat REAL food, which means food that does not come in a box or with a label. It's simpler that we make it. Reach for fruit, veggies, nut, organic meats and supplement with high quality vitamins, minerals and fish oil.

Spiritual Challenge: Prayer is work. Spend some time praying for each of your family members today. Detail your specific, bold petitions in your spiral and thank the Lord for hearing your prayers.

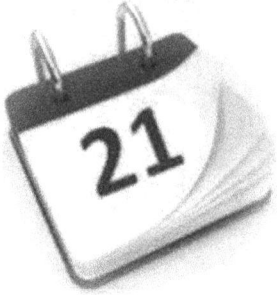

Day 21- Rest

Enjoy your day off. Play with your family. Do not do any ordinary work. Rest.

"Come to me, all who labor and are heavy laden, and I will give you rest. Take my yoke upon you, and learn from me, for I am gentle and lowly in heart, and you will find rest for your souls. For my yoke is easy, and my burden is light."

Matthew 11:28-29

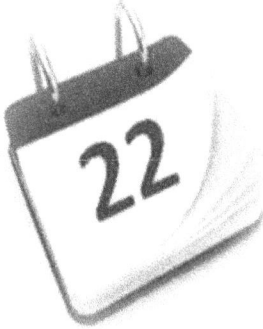

Day 22- Fat and Happy or Depleted and Tired?

In continuation from Day 20: Most people are vitamin deficient and overeat in response to the body's cry for MORE NUTRITION. Our bodies need micronutrients and if a meal does not supply the fuel it needs, it will scream for moreIso we give it more food.

Yes, that sounds like the right thing to do, but it actually leads to obesity. Unfortunately our fruits and vegetables are so depleted of nutrients that we MUST supplement, as you now know. Most people do not eat very many fruits and vegetables, anyway, therefore we MUST SUPPLEMENT.

But I want you to know that a vitamin regimen CANNOT make up for a poor diet. Your intestines will only be firm and healthy if you eat a bulky amount of vegetable fiber regularly.

And...

Your skin will only be supple and beautiful if you are hydrated from the inside out. No amount of facial lotions can make up for a poor diet.

Supplements are necessary, but they can only take you so far. Good, healthy habits must be in place if you truly want a healthy body, inside and out.

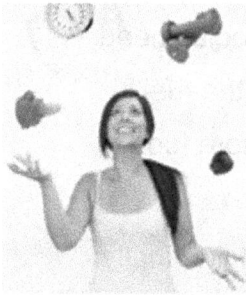

Physical Challenge: Drink herbal teas throughout the day. Different leaves have different benefits to your body, so try a variety and then buy the loose leaf in bulk. I specifically enjoy green tea and hibiscus tea. Find your favorites and sip all day long. (www.bulkherbstore.com) I also love Slique Tea by Young Living because it's yummy, boosts the metabolism and supports a healthy gut! Can't get better that! Make tea one of your fun indulgences.

Spiritual Challenge: You should be reading a chapter aloud to your kids from Proverbs each morning. This morning, take the time to memorize with your children

the verse from the chapter that speaks the loudest to you or turn it into a jingle.

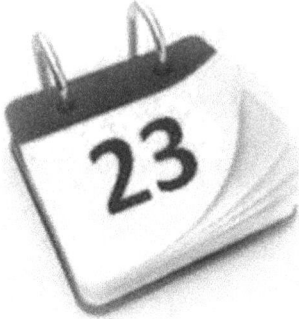

Day 23 - Breathe, Baby, Breathe

The terrified scream for help in the kitchen set me in motion. My teen vigorously patted the baby's back. The baby's eyes watered and her cheeks flushed. A quick evaluation of the scene revealed the need for CPR. Being a pro at the finger sweeping, life saving procedure, I grabbed my toddler and started to work.

However, nothing helped.

The baby would not breathe.

But there was NOTHING to dislodge. I panicked and had everyone call 911. Six cell phones dialed for help, while I ran around in circles with the baby, because that is so helpful.

It turns out that our young one had an anaphylactic reaction. My teenagers were gathered around an anomaly in our house: Chex Mix. No one noticed that our little angel reached onto the counter, while being held, and put a piece of Chex into her mouth, until she started choking.

After a teen removed the little piece, the baby still would not breathe, so the patting of her back began. The baby's body GREATLY objected to the chemicals laced on this common snack.

MSG and artificial preservatives are harmful. They not only cause heart palpitations, swelling and shortness of breath, but also memory loss. I realize that it is almost IMPOSSIBLE to go through life without EVER eating them. I just hope to persuade you to make it a rarity in your diet/a once in awhile choice. Your insides will feel cleaner and your memory sharper when you cleanse your body of preservatives.

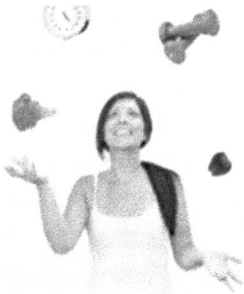

Physical Challenge: Make a cleanse part of your health routine. There are a million to choose from, but here are a few simple cleanses that I like because I'm all about simple: Digest and Cleanse capsules for daily use, The Five Day Nutritive Cleanse and The Cleansing Trio all by Young Living.

Spiritual Challenge: Cleanse the junk from your soul by forgiving those who have wronged you. Forgive them out loud. Forgive each and every one that comes to your mind that has hurt you. You will feel a heap lighter.

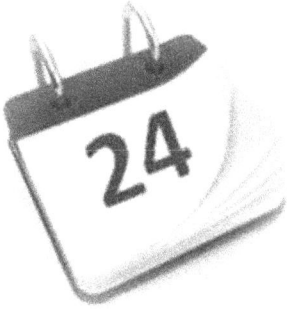

Day 24- Steady Eddie

Back up several months: The Christmas frenzy ended and I had a list of New Year's Resolutions to boot like much of the population. *Gung ho* and super excited the new year would see some fancy accomplishments by this over achiever.

Fast forward ten days and my elaborate list looked like a two-year-old's handwriting practice sheet. Most of my lofty ambitions colored out with vigorous pen scratches as real life slapped me back into reality. By January 31st ONE lone, achievable, sustainable, reasonable resolution remained.

My point is... if something is not reasonable and sustainable, it won't be sustained.

I have used the habits in 31 Days to Fit for 20ish years. They are reasonable and sustainable. You can do this. Check your list. You may be frustrated because your weight won't stabilize. The absence of ONE of these habits

COULD keep you from a boost of energy or a loss of ten pounds. I encourage you to simply apply each one of these habits for a year and I PROMISE it will make a difference in your body!

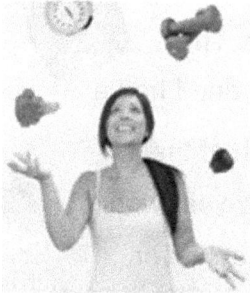

Physical Challenge: Eat breakfast. Not a lot. Just make it a habit. (I typically rotate the three following choices for breakfast: plain Greek yogurt sweetened with stevia topped with frozen mixed berries, plain organic oatmeal topped with berries, or a Slique Shake by Young Living.)

Spiritual Challenge: "..But they who wait for the Lord shall renew their strength; they shall mount up like wings like eagles; they shall run and not be weary; they shall walk and not faint," Isaiah 40:3. Write a note of encouragement to someone who has been waiting for a long time.

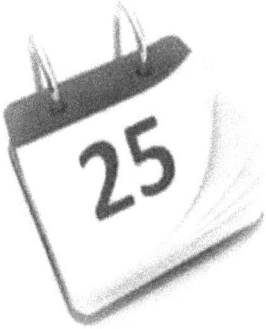

Day 25- Proper Food Combining and Enzymes!

So you have many good habits in place such as turning off the light at a decent hour, not drinking caffeine in the afternoons and walking regularly as vigorously as possible, but your body STILL DRAGS. If you feel like your energy dial is stuck on low, try proper food combining.

It is super easy, and the skip in your step after each meal will surprise you. There are some heavy laden, detail-ridden books about what should and should not be combined for proper digestion, but I am going to give you Proper Food Combining for Dummies.

It's this: Protein with veggies for one meallNO CARBS.
OR
Carbohydrates with veggieslNO PROTEIN.

Eat fruit on an empty stomach.

Pair your fat with protein, not with a carb.

In other words, separate your carbs and proteins. Do not eliminate either one of them completely from your diet. Simply allow your stomach to digest meat with veggies ALONE.

Then when you want to eat carbohydrates, combine them with veggies and NO MEAT. Your stomach uses one digestive juice to digest meat and a different one to digest carbohydrates.

Lighten the load from your stomach, and your body will return energy to your brain. Taking a digestive enzyme can also help move the food out of the stomach faster which restores energy. Enzymes can clean up plaque and eliminate old fat and proteins deposited for years. Enzymes enhance circulation and support the immune system by increasing the surface area of the red blood cell. Think healthy blood. In addition, enzymes support weight regulation, which is the reason you're reading this little book, right? You want weight regulation! It's true! This little tip could be a game changer for you! Overweight people may be lacking in lipase. In Young Living's Essentialzymes-4™, you get lipase, and in Essentialzyme, you get pancrelipase (which is a form of pancreatin that has an elevated content of lipase). The bottom line is that digestive enzymes are not optional!! You NEED THEM, even if you are using proper food combining. I properly food combine AND take Essentialzyme! If this is still fuzzy: Ask me. I would love to help you figure this out!

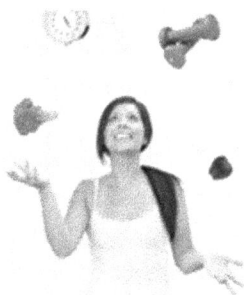

Physical Challenge: Properly combine food TODAY and you should immediately feel an energy lift. And if you suffer from stomach aches; you may get some relief. The supplement Ningxia Red gives my family an energy boost because we have found that it soothes the gut even though that's not what it's known for. Use proper food combining and study the benefits of Ningxia Red for the sake of your gut! http://ningxiared.com/benefits/

You also may need a digestive enzyme to help move your foods out. Consider Essentialzyme or Essentialzyme-4. You can read about them on the youngliving.com website.

Spiritual Challenge: Memorize: Proverbs 13:4, "The sluggard craves and gets nothing, but the desires of the diligent are fully satisfied."

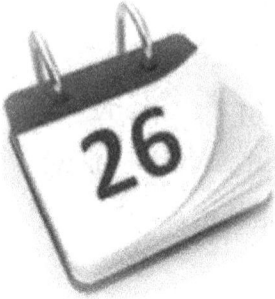

Day 26 - Too Young to Dye

Our surroundings were stunning: marble floors, beautiful light fixtures, huge windows overlooking a spouting fountain. Captivating! Yet, my little ones darted around the room in a fast game of tag like they were at the park.

They know betterland so do I. They had just filled their bellies full of bright colored sugary candy (bad idea). And in a matter of minutes hyperactivity transformed my children into little ping-pong balls.

Why on earth the FDA has approved artificial dyes is beyond me. Dyes enhance the color of candy, butter, cereals, cheese, popsicles, juice, some frozen fruit, and on and on so that we will buy these prepared items.

Studies show that dye causes behavior problems in kids, (I can attest to that) and they have been linked to cancer and general sickness. The information is easy to find on Mercola's website.

http://articles.mercola.com/sites/articles/archive/2011/04/13/the-dark-side-of-the-rainbow-of-food-dyes-being-used-to-color-your-food.aspx

Since artificial dye is almost impossible to avoid altogether, I do my best with my kids (when I'm paying attention--unlike the above example). I like to exchange it for chocolate when possible. Rather than policing the dye like a sergeant, my desire is to educate my children on the dangers of artificial color. This does not mean we will ALWAYS avoid it. One would have to live on a secluded island to achieve that!

We have discussions about the benefits of eating natural dyes found in fruits and veggies and we have mirrored the differences in natural and artificial dyes.

For instance: blueberries are extremely high in antioxidants. Antioxidants fight serious diseases. Natural dyes are powerfully good for the body. Artificial dyes are awfully dangerous to the body. Teaching your loved ones WHY they should dodge manufactured color will go much farther than simply
trying to avoid the toxins altogether.

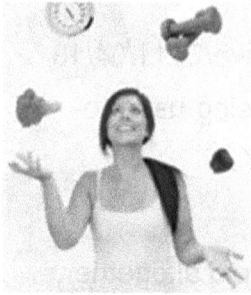

Physical Challenge: Throw away everything in your pantry and refrigerator with dye in it. I know. I know. It's the same as throwing money in the trash, but trust me. It will cost you more to cleanse the dyes out of your tissue than the food costs you. So save yourself some money in the long run and throw out the brightly colored artificial food in your house.

Spiritual Challenge: Memorize: Psalms 25:9,"He guides the humble in what is right and teaches them His way." Ask the Lord for a humble heart. Look up scriptures that contain the words humble and humility.

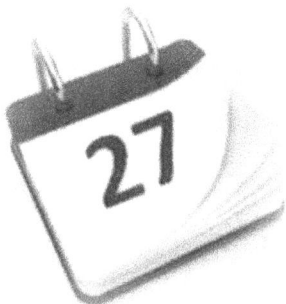

Day 27 - The Whatchamacallit

So who gives a flip about being fit if memory is a problem? Memory is an issue for many people, no matter what the age, and for a good reason. Much of the "foods" we put into our bodies chip away at our ability to remember common words, names and phrases.

I mentioned earlier that preservatives and chemicals cloud cognitive function. Caffeine also depletes the choline in the brain, which inhibits instant recall. Stress eats away the B vitamins in our cells, which also affects the way our brain works. Make a mental list of these food items that inhibit brain function and avoid them, if you can remember. Reevaluate the stress in your life for the sake of your memory.

Most of the mission statements given to me during the test run of this book, state that energy and health for the sake of maintaining vibrant family relationships are the most important reasons to stay fit. Memory falls into this category. The ability to remember the little things that are important to your loved ones will enhance your relationships: shared moments, private jokes, and special preferencesIA strong memory **trumps** being fit, but I believe you can have both!

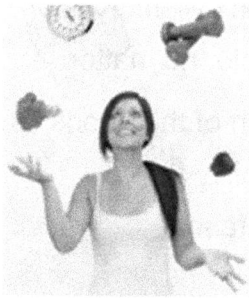

Physical Challenge: Use pure coconut oil as much as possible. Pure coconut oil has proven to strengthen brain function. Use it in place of butter in most recipes. If you desire to supplement, use Mindwise, Omegagize and or Super B. (By Young Living)

Spiritual Challenge: Memorizing scripture WILL strengthen your mind. Your memory is a muscle-- exercise it. Review each of the verses I've given you to memorize.

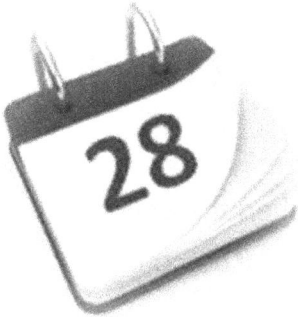

Day 28 - Rest!

"Remember the Sabbath day, to keep it holy," Exodus 20:8.

Enjoy the day off with your family!!

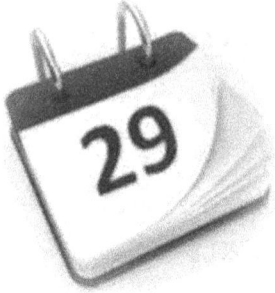

Day 29- Pass the Oil

Do you remember when the entire US got fat on Snackwells? The country went crazy eating fat free cookies, fat free ice cream, and fat free EVERYTHING! And do you remember the result?

Fat-full bottoms.

Dry skin.

Dull hair.

Slow memories.

Our bodies NEED the right type of fats to function properly, but somehow we have become a bit afraid of fat. If you will cut out the fried food and use extra virgin olive oil, coconut oil and grapeseed oil freely, you should see an overall improvement in your skin, hair, and memory.

Enjoy these God-given fats in their purest forms.

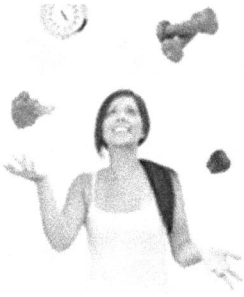

Physical Challenge: Buy avocados as often as you can. Eat them whole, put them on salads. Serve them on chicken. Enjoy them! Also, make sure you are getting AMPLE Omega 3 fatty acids everyday! This is an oil that will benefit you in many ways. When supplementing Omega fatty acids purity is of the utmost important. You don't want a source that uses dirty fish. Omegagize by Young Living meets my standard of purity.

Spiritual Challenge: Take a meal to a neighbor. Hurting people surround us: people who just need encouragement or a gesture of kindness. The deed will energize you and possibly fuel a friendship.

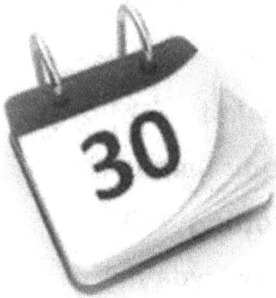

Day 30 - Ready to Fly

I hope that you have been encouraged to make a few changes or get back on the wagon in some cases. Getting and staying trim does NOT have to be complicated. These simple steps have successfully guided me through years of childbearing, nursing, raising a family and running a household. Too many women think they have to starve themselves in order to stay trim.

This simply is not true.

Eating real food in a rhythmic, balanced lifestyle will work for you. You have learned foods to avoid and foods to love. Now, learn to forgive yourself when you deem that you have *messed up.*

Every second is a new start.

Don't sabotage your progress with a giant *I'll never get this right* chocolate-eating fest. You will just feel worse afterwards. This is not a race. It is a lifestyle. You can do it. Today, review your new habits. Evaluate your progress.

Decide what your weak link is and set up a safety net to catch you. For instance, if your husband eats before bed every night and this is too tempting for you, take a shower while he snacks. Find a way to guard your goals. You can do this! I believe you can!

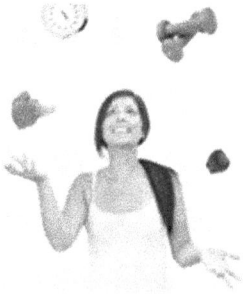

Physical Challenge: Learn to forgive yourself if you lose self- control and eat half the cheesecake. Beating yourself up for mistakes will only cause you to eat more. Stay faithful to the physical challenges above.

Spiritual Challenge: Spend time asking God to guide you into self-discipline in each area of your life. We can do so much more with the help of the Holy Spirit. Just ask.

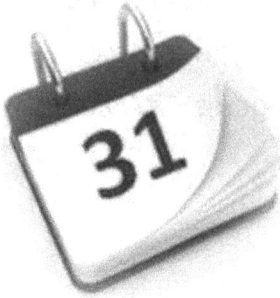

Day 31- Go!

Post this list inside your closet as a reminder of the little habits that will keep you trim for a lifetime!

1) Don't eat late.

2) Drink more water.

3) Take the stairs.

4) Walk briskly at least three times a week.

5) Eat a salad everyday.

6) Read food labels.

7) Eat frozen berries as a snack regularly.

8) Substitute raw, unbleached sugar for white, refined sugar; limit your sugar intake to two times a week. Use stevia to sweeten drinks.

9) Lift arm weights four days a week.

10) Get rid of your fat and skinny clothes. Get comfortable with your size.

11) Throw away anything in your house with artificial sweeteners.

12) Determine to eat only the recommended serving size at each meal.

13) Give up flour for 40 days.

14) Take a good multi-vitamin, Omega fish oil, and an enzyme.

15) Turn the light off at a decent hour.

16) Drink a green smoothie (almost) everyday (share with your kids!) and enjoy berry whip several times a week.

17) Eat an apple a day.

18) Eat REAL food.

19) Drink herbal teas.

20) Drink cleansing herbal tea regularly.

21) Eat breakfast.

22) Properly combine foods.

23) Throw away all the food with dye in your pantry and refrigerator.

24) Replace butter with Coconut oil as much as possible.

25) Freely eat good fats.

26) Learn to forgive yourself.

27) The five days of "Rest" in this challenge are just as important as the other habits. Don't neglect them!

Thank you for reading and God Bless!

~ Terri Bonin

justalittledrop.com

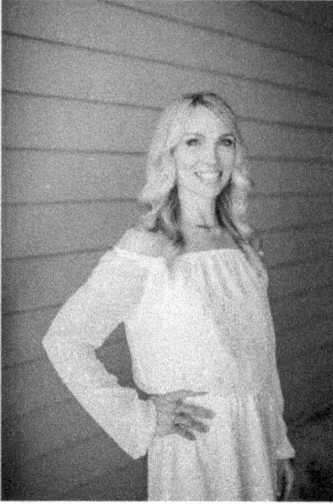

About the Author

Terri Bonin is happily married to Troy Bonin, her favorite dentist. Their union has prolifically produced eleven darling children. She has a degree in nutritional counseling, but finds she primarily uses it to persuade her children to eat their greens. When she is not juggling her daily tasks, or dating her husband, she teaches wellness classes as a means to help women grow in health education. She writes to encourage, equip and empower women to live wholeheartedly within their families.

Other books by Terri Bonin:

Drops of Pleasure: A Guide to Great Sex using Essential Oils

14 Days to Ignite Your Marriage

Live, Love, Laugh and Laundry?

Fat Proof Your Kids

A Fat Proof Meal Plan

www.ingramcontent.com/pod-product-compliance
Lightning Source LLC
Chambersburg PA
CBHW050600280326
41933CB00011B/1923